LYMPHOMA DIET PLAN COOK BOOK

The Lymphoma Diet Plan:
Delicious Dishes to Support
Lymphoma Treatment

LARRY HERMAN

Table of Contents

Introduction

A Lymphoma Diet Is A Set Of Dietary Advice Intended To Support The Overall Health And Well-Being Of Those Diagnosed With Lymphoma, Rather Than A Specific Diet Plan For Treating Or Curing The Condition. Lymphoma Is A Malignancy That Impacts The Lymphatic System, An Essential Component Of The Body's Immune System.

Although A Nutritious Diet Cannot Substitute Medical Interventions Like Chemotherapy Or Radiation Therapy, It Can Enhance Traditional Treatments And Enhance The General Health And Resilience Of Those Receiving Cancer Therapy. Consulting With Healthcare

Specialists Such As Oncologists And Registered Dietitians Is Crucial To Develop A Personalized Nutrition Plan Tailored To The Specific Needs And Problems Of An Individual's Condition And Treatment.

Here Are Some Fundamental Ideas To Consider When Discussing A Lymphoma Diet:

• Prioritize A Well-Rounded Diet Consisting Of A Mix Of Fruits, Vegetables, Whole Grains, Lean Meats, And Healthy Fats For Balanced Nutrition. Proper Diet Is Essential For Sustaining Energy, Bolstering The Immune System, And Enhancing General Health.

• Hydration Is Crucial, Particularly While Undergoing Cancer Therapy. Water Aids In Body Functioning, Promotes Digestion, And Can Relieve Side Effects Like Nausea From Therapies.

• Adequate Protein Intake Is Crucial For Preserving Muscle Mass And Facilitating The Repair Process. Lean Protein Sources Consist Of Poultry, Fish, Beans, Lentils, And Dairy Products.

• **Nutrients:** Vitamins And Minerals Concentrate On Acquiring Crucial Vitamins And Minerals From A Diverse Range Of Food Sources. This May Involve Consuming Fruits And Vegetables High In Vitamins, Obtaining

Calcium From Dairy Or Fortified Plant-Based Sources, And Acquiring Other Micronutrients Essential For Immunological Function.

• Consume Fiber-Rich Meals Such As Whole Grains, Fruits, And Vegetables To Promote Digestive Health. Individuals With Digestive Problems Due To Therapy Should Seek Advice From A Healthcare Practitioner For Tailored Instructions.

• **Personalized Approach:** Individuals' Reactions To Cancer Treatment And Dietary Requirements Can Differ. It Is Essential To Collaborate With Healthcare Professionals, Such As A Certified Dietitian, To Customize Nutritional

Advice According To Individual Health Condition, Treatment Regimen, And Particular Side Effects.

A Nutritious Diet Is Essential For Overall Well-Being But Is Not A Replacement For Medical Care. Patients Must Adhere To Their Healthcare Team's Recommendations And Consult Their Medical Specialists Regarding Any Dietary Modifications Or Supplements.

CHAPTER ONE
Fundamentals of a Lymphoma Diet

A Lymphoma Diet Focuses On Following A Nutrition Plan That Promotes General Well-Being, Sustains Energy Levels, And Manages Possible Side Effects Of Lymphoma Therapies. Here Are Some Overarching Principles:

• Follow A Balanced Diet By Including A Variety Of Colored Fruits And Vegetables To Provide A Diverse Intake Of Nutrients.

• Include Nutritious Grains Like Brown Rice, Quinoa, And Whole Wheat For A Rich Source Of Fiber And Long-Lasting Energy.

Include Lean Proteins Such As Poultry, Fish, Tofu, Lentils, And Low-Fat Dairy In Your Diet.

- **Hydration:** Maintain Proper Hydration By Consuming Ample Water Throughout The Day. Ensuring Adequate Hydration Can Assist In Controlling Side Effects Such As Nausea And Promoting General Well-Being.

- Consume Moderate Amounts Of Healthy Fats Such As Avocados, Nuts, Seeds, And Olive Oil. Avoid Consuming Saturated And Trans Fats Commonly Included In Processed Foods And Fried Goods.

• Consume Protein-Rich Foods With Every Meal To Promote Muscular Strength And Aid In Repair. Excellent Sources Comprise Lean Meats, Chicken, Fish, Eggs, Dairy, Beans, And Legumes.

• Eating Small, Frequent Meals Might Help Control Appetite And Reduce Nausea, Particularly During Or After Treatments.

• Choose Nutrient-Dense Snacks Like Fresh Fruits, Veggies With Hummus, Yogurt, Or Almonds To Boost Energy Levels Between Meals.

• Avoid Consuming Processed Foods, Sugary Snacks, And Sugary Beverages As Much As Possible. These

Substances Can Cause Inflammation and Lack Necessary Nutrients.

• Discuss The Utilization Of Dietary Supplements, Like Vitamins And Minerals, With Healthcare Specialists To Address Possible Deficiencies. Supplements Should Not Be Used As A Substitute For A Well-Rounded Diet.

• Customize The Diet According To Individual Requirements And Tolerances. Individuals May Have Alterations In Taste, Appetite, Or Gastrointestinal Problems While Undergoing Therapy, Necessitating Adjustments To Their Diet.

• Seek Guidance From Healthcare Specialists, Such As Oncologists And

Qualified Dietitians, Before Making Substantial Dietary Modifications. They Can Offer Tailored Suggestions According To The Particular Lymphoma Kind, Treatment Regimen, And Personal Health Condition.

The Dietary Requirements For Individuals With Lymphoma Can Vary, And The Instructions Provided Are Basic Principles. Patients Should Collaborate With Their Healthcare Team To Create A Customized Nutrition Plan Tailored To Their Individual Circumstances, Therapy, And Any Adverse Effects.

The Significance of Nutrition in Lymphoma Treatment

Nutrition Is Vital In Aiding Those Receiving Cancer Treatment. It Is Crucial To Maintain A Well-Rounded And Healthy Diet For Various Reasons In The Current Hard Circumstances.

• Coping With Lymphoma Treatment Effects: - Chemotherapy And Radiation Therapy For Lymphoma Can Be Strenuous And Cause Fatigue. Sufficient Nourishment Sustains Energy Levels, Aiding The Body In Managing The Requirements Of Treatment.

• **Enhancing the Immune System:** The Immune System Is Crucial In Protecting The Body Against Cancer

Cells. Optimal Nutrition Is Crucial For Bolstering Immune Function, Combating Infections, And Facilitating The Recovery Process.

• **Maintaining Muscular Mass:** Cancer Therapies May Result In Muscular Atrophy And Weight Reduction. Sufficient Protein Consumption Is Essential For Maintaining Muscle Mass, Supporting Recovery, And Avoiding Malnutrition.

• Treatment Side Effects Of Lymphoma Can Be Managed And Alleviated By Nutrition. An Effectively Planned Diet Can Alleviate Nausea, Promote Digestive Well-Being, And Manage Alterations In Appetite Or Taste.

• **Promoting Healing And Recovery:**
Adequate Nutrition Is Essential For Tissue Regeneration And Recuperation. It Can Expedite The Recovery Process From Treatments, Surgeries, Or Other Medical Procedures.

• Proper Diet Might Decrease The Likelihood Of Infections, Which Is A Worry For Those With Weakened Immune Systems From Cancer Therapies.

• **Enhancing Quality Of Life:** Optimal Nutrition Enhances The Body's Ability To Manage The Physical And Emotional Strain Of Cancer Therapy. It Can Have A Beneficial Effect On The

Overall Quality Of Life Both During And After Therapy.

- **Managing Treatment-Related Anemia:** Anemia May Occur In Certain Persons Receiving Lymphoma Treatment. Sufficient Consumption Of Iron And Vitamin B12, In Addition To Other Essential Nutrients, Can Assist In Controlling And Preventing Anemia.

- **Improving Tolerance To Treatment:** Individuals Who Are Well-Nourished May Have Enhanced Tolerance To Cancer Therapies. This Can Lead To More Efficient Fulfillment Of Treatment Goals.

- Psychological Well-Being Can Be Improved By Eating Well, Which Can

Help Individuals Feel A Sense Of Control And Well-Being During Difficult Times.

The Nutritional Requirements For Individuals With Lymphoma Can Differ, And A Universal Strategy May Not Be Suitable. It Is Advisable To Collaborate With Healthcare Professionals Such As Oncologists And Registered Dietitians To Create A Customized Nutrition Plan Tailored To The Specific Type Of Lymphoma, Individual Health Condition, And Treatment Regimen. This Collaborative Approach Guarantees That The Dietary Suggestions Are Tailored To The Specific Needs And Circumstances Of Each Patient.

CHAPTER TWO
Essential Nutrients for Individuals with Lymphoma

Lymphoma Patients Can Benefit From A Balanced Diet That Supplies Critical Nutrients To Enhance General Health, Strengthen Immunity, And Address Any Treatment Adverse Effects. Key Nutrients Essential For Lymphoma Treatment:

• Protein Is Vital For The Maintenance And Regeneration Of Tissues, Particularly Muscles, Which Is Critical During Cancer Treatment.

• Sources Include Lean Meats, Poultry, Fish, Eggs, Dairy Products, Legumes, Nuts, And Seeds.

• Calories Are Essential For Sustaining Energy Levels, Particularly When Addressing Potential Weight Loss And Weariness.

• Sources Include Whole Grains, Lean Proteins, Healthy Fats, Fruits, And Vegetables.

• Fiber Is Essential For Promoting Gut Health And Can Aid In Relieving Constipation, A Frequent Complication Of Several Cancer Therapies.

• Sources Include Whole Grains, Fruits, Vegetables, Legumes, And Nuts.

• Antioxidants Are Crucial For Safeguarding Cells Against Harm From Free Radicals, Which May Lower The

Chances Of Difficulties And Promote General Well-Being.

- **Sources:** Vibrantly Colored Fruits And Vegetables Include Berries, Oranges, Spinach, And Broccoli.

- Vitamins And Minerals Are Crucial For Multiple Biological Processes, Such As Immune System Support, Bone Strength, And Overall Wellness.

- Sources Of Vitamin C Include Citrus Fruits, Strawberries, And Bell Peppers.

- Vitamin D Sources Include Fatty Fish, Fortified Dairy Products, And Exposure To Sunlight.

- Calcium Sources Include Dairy Products, Fortified Plant-Based Milk, And Leafy Greens.

• Iron Can Be Found In Lean Meats, Beans, Lentils, And Fortified Cereals.

• Folate Sources Include Leafy Greens, Legumes, And Fortified Grains.

• B Vitamins Can Be Found In Whole Grains, Meat, Fish, And Dairy Products.

• **Omega-3 Fatty Acids:** Significance: Can Exhibit Anti-Inflammatory Properties And Promote Cardiovascular Health.

• Sources Of Omega-3 Fatty Acids Include Fatty Fish (Salmon, Mackerel, Sardines), Flaxseeds, Chia Seeds, And Walnuts.

• Fluids Are Crucial For Preventing Dehydration, Particularly During

Cancer Therapies To Alleviate Potential Side Effects Such As Nausea.

- Sources Of Hydration Include Water, Herbal Teas, Broths, And Hydrating Fruits And Vegetables.

- Consuming Small, Frequent Meals Might Assist With Appetite Control And Reduce Nausea, Which Are Sometimes Experienced During Therapy.

- Sources of Nutrients: Nutrient-Dense Foods Such As Fresh Fruits, Veggies with Hummus, Yogurt, and Almonds.

- Adaptogens Are Herbs That Can Assist The Body In Adapting To Stress And Promoting General Well-Being.

Consult Healthcare Specialists Before Using Adaptogens, Such As Plants Like Ashwagandha Or Holy Basil.

• Collaborating With Healthcare Specialists, Such As Oncologists And Certified Dietitians, Is Essential For Tailored Assistance, Addressing Individual Needs, And Managing Potential Treatment Interactions.

Lymphoma Patients Should Collaborate Closely With Healthcare Specialists To Customize Their Diet According To Their Unique Circumstances, Treatment Regimen, And Possible Side Effects, As Individual Nutritional Requirements Can Differ. Customized Advice Guarantees That Dietary Suggestions

Are In Accordance With Specific Health Objectives And General Welfare.

Designing a Lymphoma-Focused Meal Plan

To Create A Lymphoma-Focused Meal Plan, One Must Design A Well-Balanced And Nutritious Diet That Promotes General Health, Manages Treatment Side Effects, And Supplies Essential Nutrients For Recovery. It Is Essential To Engage With Healthcare Specialists, Particularly A Qualified Dietitian, To Customize The Strategy According To Individual Needs. Here Is A Basic Outline For Creating A Meal Plan Focusing On Lymphoma.

1. **Base The Diet On Whole Foods:**
Prioritize Whole, Minimally Processed Foods To Ensure A Diverse Range Of Nutrients.

2. **Balanced Macronutrients:**

- **Protein:** Include Lean Proteins Like Poultry, Fish, Eggs, Tofu, Legumes, And Low-Fat Dairy.

- **Carbohydrates:** Choose Whole Grains (Brown Rice, Quinoa, Whole Wheat), Fruits, And Vegetables For Sustained Energy.

- **Fats:** Opt For Healthy Fats From Avocados, Nuts, Seeds, And Olive Oil.

3. **Fruits and Vegetables:** Aim for a Variety of Colorful Fruits And Vegetables To Provide Antioxidants, Vitamins, And Minerals.

- Incorporate Dark Leafy Greens, Berries, Citrus Fruits, And Cruciferous Vegetables.

4. **Hydration:** Drink Plenty Of Water Throughout The Day To Stay Hydrated, Especially Important During Treatment.

5. **Small, Frequent Meals:** Consider Smaller, More Frequent Meals To Manage Appetite And Prevent Nausea.

Include Nutrient-Dense Snacks Like Yogurt With Fruit, Whole-Grain Crackers With Hummus, Or Nuts.

6. **Probiotics And Digestive Health:** Include Probiotic-Rich Foods Like Yogurt Or Kefir To Support Gut Health, Which Can Be Affected By Treatment.

7. **Fiber-Rich Foods:** Incorporate Fiber From Whole Grains, Fruits, Vegetables, And Legumes To Support Digestive Health.

8. **Omega-3 Fatty Acids:** Include Fatty Fish (Salmon, Mackerel), Flaxseeds, Chia Seeds, Or Walnuts For Anti-Inflammatory Effects.

9. **Supplementation:** Discuss The Need For Supplements (Vitamins, Minerals) With Healthcare Professionals To Address Potential Deficiencies.

10. **Adapt To Taste Changes:** If Taste Changes Are Experienced, Experiment With Different Seasonings And Cooking Methods To Make Food More Appealing.

• Cold Or Room Temperature Foods May Be Better Tolerated If Sensitivity To Hot Foods Is An Issue.

11. **Avoid Certain Foods:** If Specific Foods Cause Discomfort Or Worsen Side Effects, Consider Avoiding Them Temporarily.

• Limit Processed Foods, Sugary Snacks, And Foods High In Saturated Fats.

12. **Collaborate With Healthcare Team:** Regularly Communicate With Healthcare Professionals To Adjust The Meal Plan Based On Individual Needs, Treatment Responses, And Side Effects.

Sample Day:

Breakfast:

- Oatmeal with Berries and a Sprinkle of Flaxseeds.
- Greek Yogurt with Honey and Walnuts.

Snack:

- Apple Slices with Almond Butter.

Lunch:

- Grilled Chicken or Tofu Salad with Mixed Greens, Cherry Tomatoes, and Quinoa.
- Whole-Grain Roll.

Snack:

• Carrot Sticks With Hummus.

Dinner:

- Baked Salmon or Lentil Stew.
- Steamed Broccoli and Brown Rice.

Dessert:

• Fresh Fruit Salad.

This Is A Broad Guidance, Individual Needs May Differ. Always Seek

Guidance From Healthcare Professionals For Tailored Recommendations Depending On The Exact Form Of Lymphoma, Treatment Regimen, And Individual Health Condition.

CHAPTER THREE
Foods to Include In a Lymphoma Diet

A Lymphoma Diet Should Consist Of Diverse Range Of Nutrient-Dense Foods To Enhance General Well-Being, Strengthen The Immune System, And Address Any Treatment-Related Side Effects. Here Is A List Of Foods To Consider Including:

1. Lean Proteins:

- Skinless Poultry (Chicken, Turkey)
- Fish (Salmon, Trout, Tuna)
- Lean Cuts Of Beef Or Pork
- Tofu, Tempeh, And Other Plant-Based Proteins

- Beans And Legumes (Lentils, Chickpeas, Black Beans)
- Low-Fat Dairy Products (Yogurt, Cottage Cheese)

2. Colorful Fruits:

- Berries (Blueberries, Strawberries, Raspberries)
- Citrus Fruits (Oranges, Grapefruits)
- Apples, Pears, And Stone Fruits (Peaches, Plums)
- Kiwi, Pineapple, Mango
- Tomatoes (Technically A Fruit)

3. Vibrant Vegetables:

- Dark Leafy Greens (Spinach, Kale, Swiss Chard)

- Cruciferous Vegetables (Broccoli, Cauliflower, Brussels Sprouts)
- Carrots, Sweet Potatoes, And Winter Squash
- Bell Peppers (Red, Yellow, Green)
- Colorful Root Vegetables (Beets, Turnips, Radishes)

4. Whole Grains:

- Brown Rice, Wild Rice
- Quinoa, Bulgur, Barley
- Whole Wheat Pasta And Bread
- Oats And Oatmeal
- Millet, Amaranth, Farro

5. Healthy Fats:

- Avocado

- Nuts And Seeds (Almonds, Walnuts, Chia Seeds, Flaxseeds)
- Olive Oil, Avocado Oil
- Fatty Fish (Salmon, Mackerel, Sardines)
- Nut Butters (Peanut Butter, Almond Butter)

6. Dairy and Dairy Alternatives:

- Low-Fat Milk Or Fortified Plant-Based Milk (Soy, Almond, Oat)
- Greek Yogurt Or Dairy-Free Yogurt Alternatives
- Cheese (In Moderation)

7. Herbs, Spices, and Flavorings:

- Fresh Herbs (Parsley, Cilantro, Basil)

- Spices (Turmeric, Ginger, Cinnamon, Cumin)
- Garlic, Onions, Shallots
- Lemon Or Lime Juice
- Vinegars (Balsamic, Apple Cider)

8. Hydrating Foods:

- Cucumbers
- Watermelon
- Celery
- Oranges
- Soups And Broths

9. Probiotic-Rich Foods:

- Yogurt (With Live And Active Cultures)
- Kefir

- Fermented Vegetables (Sauerkraut, Kimchi)

10. High-Fiber Foods:

- Whole Grains (Oats, Quinoa, Brown Rice)
- Fruits (Apples, Berries, Pears)
- Vegetables (Broccoli, Brussels Sprouts, Carrots)
- Legumes (Beans, Lentils, Chickpeas)

11. Fluids:

- Water
- Herbal Teas
- Coconut Water
- Clear Broths

12. Nutrient-Dense Snacks:

- Fresh Fruit Slices Or Whole Fruit

- Raw Vegetable Sticks With Hummus Or Guacamole

- Greek Yogurt With Honey And Nuts

- Trail Mix With Nuts, Seeds, And Dried Fruit

- Rice Cakes With Almond Butter Or Avocado

13. Considerations:

• Individual Tolerances And Preferences May Vary. Experiment With Different Foods To Find What Works Best For You.

• Avoid Foods That Cause Discomfort or Exacerbate Side Effects, Such As

Spicy Foods Or Foods High In Sugar And Saturated Fats.

• Consult With Healthcare Professionals, Including A Registered Dietitian, For Personalized Recommendations Based On Your Specific Needs And Circumstances.

Incorporating Diverse Range Of Nutrient-Dense Foods Into Your Diet Will Help Maintain Your General Health And Well-Being While Dealing With Lymphoma And Its Therapies.

Avoid These Foods

When Creating A Diet For Those Receiving Cancer Therapies, It's Crucial To Consider Specific Foods That Could Worsen Side Effects Or Hinder Nutritional Objectives. Dietary Guidelines May Differ Depending On Individual Tolerances And Preferences. Seeking Guidance From Healthcare Specialists, Such As A Qualified Dietitian, Is Essential For Tailored Recommendations. Here Are Some General Tips On Foods To Avoid Or Limit During Cancer Treatment:

1. Highly Processed Foods:

- Processed Snacks (Chips, Cookies, Candy)
- Fast Food And Fried Foods

- Sugary Cereals And Pastries

2. Sugary Foods and Beverages:

- Candy, Sweets, And Desserts With Added Sugars
- Sugary Beverages (Sodas, Fruit Juices With Added Sugar)
- Excessive Consumption Of Sugary Snacks

3. High-Fat and Greasy Foods:

- Fried Foods
- Fatty Cuts Of Meat
- Foods High In Saturated And Trans Fats

4. Spicy Foods:

- Spicy Dishes May Exacerbate Digestive Issues Or Irritation,

Especially If Experiencing Mouth Sores Or Gastrointestinal Discomfort.

5. Foods High In Salt:

- Processed and Salty Snacks
- Canned And Processed Foods With High Sodium Content
- Limiting Salt May Help Manage Fluid Retention And High Blood Pressure.

6. Raw or Undercooked Foods:

• To Reduce The Risk Of Foodborne Illnesses, Especially If The Immune System Is Compromised, Avoid Raw Or Undercooked Meats, Eggs, And Seafood.

7. Acidic Foods:

- Citrus Fruits And Juices (Oranges, Grapefruits)
- Tomatoes And Tomato-Based Products
- Limiting Acidic Foods May Be Beneficial For Individuals Experiencing Mouth Sores Or Acid Reflux.

8. Alcohol:

- Alcohol Can Interact With Medications And Compromise Liver Function. It's Generally Advisable To Limit Or Avoid Alcohol During Treatment.

9. Large Meals:

• Instead Of Consuming Large Meals, Consider Smaller, More Frequent Meals To Manage Nausea And Promote Better Digestion.

10. Dairy If Lactose Intolerant:

• For Individuals Who Are Lactose Intolerant, Dairy Products May Cause Digestive Discomfort. Consider Lactose-Free Alternatives.

11. Individual Allergens Or Sensitivities:

• Avoid Foods That Trigger Allergies Or Sensitivities. Common Allergens Include Gluten, Nuts, Shellfish, And Soy.

12. Personal Preferences And Tolerances:

• Individual Preferences And Tolerances Vary. Pay Attention To How Your Body Responds To Certain Foods And Adjust Your Diet Accordingly.

13. Consult With Healthcare Professionals:

• Always Consult With Healthcare Professionals, Including A Registered Dietitian, Before Making Significant Changes To Your Diet. They Can Provide Personalized Recommendations Based On Your Specific Health Status And Treatment Plan.

It Is Essential To Keep Transparent Communication With Your Healthcare Team To Discuss Any Issues Or Alterations In Your Dietary Requirements. Customized Dietary Guidance Is Tailored To Your Specific Health Objectives And Conditions While Undergoing Cancer Therapy.

CHAPTER FOUR
Hydration and Its Importance

Hydration Is The Act Of Ensuring The Body Has Sufficient Fluid Levels, Which Is Crucial For General Health And Welfare. Proper Hydration Is Vital For Those Receiving Lymphoma Treatment Due To Various Causes.

1. Supports Overall Health: Hydration Is Vital For Maintaining Essential Bodily Functions, Including Regulating Body Temperature, Supporting Digestion, And Transporting Nutrients And Oxygen To Cells.

2. Helps Manage Side Effects: Adequate Hydration Can Help Manage Common Side Effects Of Lymphoma Treatment, Such As Nausea, Vomiting, Diarrhea, And Mouth Sores. It Can Also Alleviate Symptoms Of Dehydration, Such As Dizziness And Fatigue.

3. Supports Kidney Function: Proper Hydration Supports Kidney Function By Helping To Flush Out Waste Products And Toxins From The Body. This Is Especially Important During Treatment When The Kidneys May Be Under Additional Stress.

4. Improves Skin Health: Hydration Plays A Key Role In Maintaining Skin Health And Elasticity. Drinking Enough Fluids Can Help Prevent

Dryness And Promote Healthy-Looking Skin, Which May Be Affected By Cancer Treatments.

5. Reduces The Risk Of Infections: Staying Hydrated Supports The Body's Immune System, Reducing The Risk Of Infections, Which Is Important For Individuals With Compromised Immune Systems Due To Cancer Treatments.

6. Supports Energy Levels: Dehydration Can Lead To Feelings Of Fatigue And Weakness. By Staying Adequately Hydrated, Individuals Undergoing Lymphoma Treatment Can Maintain Energy Levels And Better Cope With The Physical Demands Of Therapy.

7. Enhances Treatment Tolerance:
Proper Hydration Can Improve Tolerance To Cancer Treatments, Such As Chemotherapy And Radiation Therapy. It May Help Minimize Treatment Interruptions And Support Overall Treatment Effectiveness.

8. Aids in Nutrient Absorption:
Hydration Is Essential For Proper Nutrient Absorption In The Digestive Tract. Drinking Enough Fluids Ensures That Nutrients From Food Are Effectively Absorbed And Utilized By The Body.

9. Prevents Electrolyte Imbalance:
Electrolytes, Such As Sodium, Potassium, And Magnesium, Are Essential For Various Bodily

Functions. Proper Hydration Helps Maintain Electrolyte Balance, Which Is Crucial For Heart Health, Muscle Function, And Nerve Transmission.

10. Improves Mood And Cognitive Function: Dehydration Can Impair Cognitive Function And Mood, Leading To Decreased Concentration, Irritability, And Headaches. Staying Hydrated Supports Mental Clarity And Emotional Well-Being.

Tips for Hydration:

• Drink Water Regularly Throughout The Day, Aiming For At Least 8 Glasses (64 Ounces) Per Day, Or More If Recommended By Healthcare Professionals.

• Consider Hydrating Foods Such As Fruits, Vegetables, Soups, And Broths.

• Limit Or Avoid Caffeinated And Alcoholic Beverages, As They Can Contribute To Dehydration.

• Monitor Urine Color; Pale Yellow Or Straw-Colored Urine Indicates Adequate Hydration.

• Stay Hydrated Before, During, And After Lymphoma Treatments To Help Mitigate Side Effects And Support Recovery.

Emphasizing The Importance Of Being Hydrated In A Holistic Care Regimen Can Help People Receiving Lymphoma Therapy Improve Their Well-Being,

Treatment Effectiveness, And Quality Of Life.

Unique Considerations for Patients with Lymphoma

Lymphoma Patients Need Specific Dietary And Nutritional Attention Because Of The Distinct Problems Presented By The Disease And Its Therapies. Here Are Some Important Factors To Consider:

1. Immune Support: Lymphoma And Its Treatments Can Weaken The Immune System, Making Patients More Susceptible To Infections. Focus On Immune-Supportive Foods Rich In Vitamins, Minerals, And Antioxidants, Such As Fruits, Vegetables, And Lean Proteins.

2. Digestive Health: Some Lymphoma Treatments, Such As Chemotherapy And Radiation Therapy, Can Cause Gastrointestinal Side Effects Like Nausea, Vomiting, Diarrhea, And Mouth Sores. Opt For Bland, Easy-To-Digest Foods And Stay Hydrated. Avoid Spicy, Greasy, Or Acidic Foods That May Exacerbate Symptoms.

3. Nutritional Needs: Lymphoma Treatments May Affect Appetite, Leading To Changes In Food Preferences And Weight Loss. Prioritize Nutrient-Dense Foods To Meet Nutritional Needs, Including Lean Proteins, Whole Grains, Fruits, And Vegetables. Consider Smaller,

More Frequent Meals If Appetite Is Reduced.

4. Hydration: Adequate Hydration Is Crucial For Lymphoma Patients, Especially During Treatments. Drink Plenty Of Fluids, Including Water, Herbal Teas, And Hydrating Foods Like Fruits And Soups, To Prevent Dehydration And Support Overall Health.

5. Anemia Management: Some Lymphoma Patients May Experience Anemia Due To Cancer-Related Factors Or Treatments. Include Iron-Rich Foods Such As Lean Meats, Poultry, Fish, Beans, Lentils, Fortified Cereals, And Leafy Greens To Support Red Blood Cell Production.

6. Bone Health: Certain Lymphoma Treatments, Such As Corticosteroids And Radiation Therapy, Can Increase The Risk Of Osteoporosis And Bone Fractures. Consume Foods Rich In Calcium And Vitamin D, Such As Dairy Products, Fortified Plant-Based Milk, Leafy Greens, And Fatty Fish, To Support Bone Health.

7. Side Effect Management: Work Closely With Healthcare Professionals, Including Oncologists And Registered Dietitians, To Manage Treatment-Related Side Effects. They Can Provide Personalized Dietary Recommendations And Strategies To Alleviate Symptoms Like Nausea, Taste Changes, And Mouth Sores.

8. Immunosuppression Precautions:
Lymphoma Patients May Be
Immunosuppressed Due To
Treatments Like Chemotherapy. Take
Precautions To Minimize The Risk Of
Foodborne Illnesses, Such As Washing
Hands Thoroughly, Practicing Proper
Food Safety And Hygiene, And
Avoiding Raw Or Undercooked Foods.

9. Individualized Approach: Every
Lymphoma Patient's Nutritional Needs
And Tolerances Are Unique. Consider
Individual Preferences, Cultural
Considerations, And Dietary
Restrictions When Designing A
Personalized Nutrition Plan. Regularly
Assess And Adjust The Diet Based On

Treatment Responses And Evolving Needs.

10. Emotional Support: Coping With A Lymphoma Diagnosis And Its Treatments Can Be Emotionally Challenging. Seek Support From Healthcare Professionals, Support Groups, Or Mental Health Professionals As Needed. Emotional Well-Being Is An Integral Part Of Overall Health And Recovery.

By Addressing These Special Considerations And Adopting A Comprehensive Approach To Nutrition And Dietary Management, Lymphoma Patients Can Optimize Their Health, Support Treatment Outcomes, And

Improve Their Quality Of Life
Throughout Their Cancer Journey.

CHAPTER FIVE
Recipes for a Lymphoma Diet

When Creating Meals For A Lymphoma Diet, Prioritize Nutrient-Rich, Easily Digestible, And Well-Tolerated Foods. Here Are Two Basic Dishes That Include A Range Of Nutritious Foods Acceptable For People Receiving Lymphoma Treatment:

1. Quinoa and Vegetable Stir-Fry:

Ingredients:

- 1 Cup Quinoa (Rinsed And Cooked According To Package Instructions)
- 1 Tablespoon Olive Oil
- 1 Cup Broccoli Florets

- 1 Bell Pepper, Thinly Sliced

- 1 Carrot, Julienned

- 1 Zucchini, Sliced

- 2 Cloves Garlic, Minced

- 1 Tablespoon Low-Sodium Soy Sauce

- 1 Teaspoon Sesame Oil

- 1 Teaspoon Grated Ginger

- Sesame Seeds For Garnish

- Fresh Cilantro For Garnish

Instructions:

1. Cook Quinoa According To Package Instructions and Set Aside.

2. In A Large Skillet or Wok, Heat Olive Oil over Medium-High Heat.

3. Add Garlic And Ginger, Sauté For 1-2 Minutes Until Fragrant.

4. Add Broccoli, Bell Pepper, Carrot, And Zucchini To The Skillet. Stir-Fry Until Vegetables Are Tender-Crisp.

5. Add Cooked Quinoa to the Skillet and Stir Well.

6. Drizzle Soy Sauce and Sesame Oil over the Mixture. Toss Until Everything Is Evenly Coated.

7. Garnish with Sesame Seeds and Fresh Cilantro before Serving.

2. Creamy Butternut Squash Soup:

Ingredients:

- 1 Medium-Sized Butternut Squash, Peeled, Seeded, And Diced
- 1 Tablespoon Olive Oil
- 1 Onion, Diced
- 2 Carrots, Peeled And Chopped
- 2 Celery Stalks, Chopped
- 2 Cloves Garlic, Minced
- 4 Cups Low-Sodium Vegetable Broth
- 1 Teaspoon Ground Turmeric
- 1/2 Teaspoon Ground Ginger
- Salt And Pepper To Taste
- 1/2 Cup Coconut Milk (Light)
- Fresh Parsley For Garnish

Instructions:

1. In A Large Pot, Heat Olive Oil Over Medium Heat. Add Onions, Carrots, Celery, And Garlic. Sauté Until Vegetables Are Softened.

2. Add Diced Butternut Squash, Turmeric, Ginger, Salt, And Pepper. Stir To Combine.

3. Pour In The Vegetable Broth And Bring The Mixture To A Boil. Reduce Heat And Simmer Until The Squash Is Tender.

4. Use An Immersion Blender To Puree The Soup Until Smooth. Alternatively, Transfer To A Blender In Batches And Blend Until Smooth.

5. Stir In Coconut Milk and Adjust Seasoning If Necessary.

6. Garnish with Fresh Parsley before Serving.

These Recipes Emphasize The Inclusion Of A Diverse Range Of Colorful Veggies, Lean Proteins, And Whole Grains To Offer Vital Nutrients. Customize The Recipes According To Personal Preferences And Dietary Restrictions, And Seek Advice From Healthcare Professionals For Tailored Recommendations.

The Significance Of Physical Activity

Physical Activity Is Essential For General Health And Well-Being, And It Is Particularly Important For Persons Receiving Cancer Treatment. Regular Physical Activity Has Several Advantages, Particularly While Undergoing Cancer Treatment. Here Are Some Primary Reasons Why Physical Activity Is Crucial:

1. Regular Exercise Helps Preserve And Enhance Muscle Strength, Flexibility, And Overall Physical Fitness. It Is Crucial During And After Lymphoma Treatments, As They Might Cause Weariness And Muscle Weakness.

2. Boosts Energy Levels:

• Engaging In Physical Activity Has Been Proven To Decrease Tiredness And Enhance Energy Levels. Despite The Difficulties Of Cancer Treatments, Including Low-Impact Workouts Like Walking Or Yoga Can Help Boost Energy Levels.

3. Enhances Immune Function:

• Engaging In Regular Physical Activity Is Linked To Enhanced Immune Function. It Is Essential For Persons With Lymphoma To Prioritize Having A Robust Immune System, Particularly When Undergoing Treatments That Could Weaken Immune Function.

4. Assists In Managing Treatment Side Effects:

• Exercise Can Aid In Managing Typical Side Effects Of Cancer Therapies Such As Nausea, Constipation, And Sleep Difficulties. It May Also Enhance Mood And Alleviate Anxiety.

5. Manages Stress And Enhances Mental Health:

• Engaging In Physical Activity Effectively Reduces Stress And Boosts Mood. Exercise Triggers The Release Of Endorphins, Which Are The Body's Natural Mood Enhancers, And Can Alleviate Anxiety And Despair Sometimes Associated With Cancer Treatment.

6. Facilitates Weight Management:

• Maintaining A Healthy Weight Is Crucial For General Well-Being. Engaging In Physical Activity And Maintaining A Balanced Diet Can Assist In Controlling Body Weight And Avoiding Significant Weight Fluctuations While Undergoing Treatment.

7. Enhances Cardiovascular Health:

Engaging In Cardiovascular Activities Like Brisk Walking Or Cycling Supports Heart Health. It Is Crucial For Persons Receiving Lymphoma Treatment To Be Aware That Certain Medicines Can Impact The Cardiovascular System.

8. Enhances Sleep Quality: Regular Physical Activity Can Improve Sleep Quality, Which Is Crucial For General Recovery And Well-Being.

9. Improves Bone Health: Weight-Bearing Workouts Like Walking And Resistance Training Support Bone Health. This Is Especially Important For Persons Receiving Medications That Could Impact Bone Density.

Individuals With Lymphoma Should Consult Their Healthcare Team Before Starting Or Changing An Exercise Regimen. Physical Exercise Should Be Customized To Fit The Individual's Unique Situation, And Any Issues Or Restrictions Should Be Addressed With Healthcare Specialists.

Conclusion

Ultimately, A Thorough And Tailored Strategy For Handling Lymphoma Is Crucial For Maximizing The Health And Quality Of Life Of Patients During Their Treatment Process. This Strategy Includes Aspects Such As Nutrition, Hydration, Physical Activity, And Emotional Support.

A Diet Focused On Lymphoma Should Emphasize Nutrient-Rich Foods Tailored To Individual Requirements And Problems Connected To Treatment. Working With Healthcare Specialists, Especially Licensed Dietitians, Guarantees That Dietary Advice Matches The Specific Needs Of Each Patient.

Proper Hydration Is Essential For Controlling Medication Adverse Effects And Maintaining Overall Health. It Is Crucial To Stay Properly Hydrated During Lymphoma Therapy To Reduce The Chances Of Dehydration And Improve Resilience.

Engaging In Physical Activity Is A Potent Tool For Enhancing Strength, Combating Weariness, And Boosting Mental Well-Being. Customizing Workout Plans Based On Individual Abilities And Preferences Enhances Feelings Of Empowerment And Has A Beneficial Impact On Treatment Results.

Providing Emotional Support Is Crucial During The Course Of Dealing

With Cancer, Recognizing The Psychological Difficulties Individuals May Encounter. Facilitating Social Contacts, Offering Counseling Services, And Nurturing A Comprehensive Support System Enhance Overall Well-Being.

A Collaborative And Comprehensive Strategy, Encompassing Healthcare Professionals, Caregivers, And Individuals, Is Essential For Negotiating The Intricacies Of Lymphoma Treatment. Patients Can Improve Their Quality Of Life, Resilience, And Recovery During And After Cancer Therapy By Addressing Their Dietary, Physical, And Emotional Needs In A Tailored Way. Consistent

Contact With Healthcare Teams Allows For Adjustments In Strategy According To Individual Reactions And Changing Situations, Leading To A More Favorable And Empowered Experience For Persons Dealing With Lymphoma.

THE END